Get fit at home

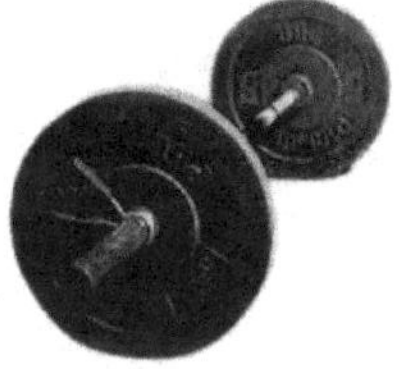

A beginner's guide to home workout

J.B. Blackwood

Table of Contents

Introduction

Emily had always dreamed of being fit and healthy, but her busy schedule and the demands of everyday life left her with little time to pursue her goal. She yearned for a way to improve her fitness without sacrificing precious hours commuting to the gym or investing in expensive exercise equipment.

One fateful day, Emily stumbled upon a magazine article that shared the remarkable stories of individuals who had transformed their lives by getting fit at home. Intrigued by their tales of success, Emily began to delve deeper into the concept of home fitness. What she discovered was a world of possibility—a world where convenience, affordability, and effectiveness converged to create a pathway to wellness right within the comfort of her own home.

Inspired by these stories, Emily embarked on her journey to become the best version of herself. With determination and a bit of resourcefulness, she transformed her living room into a vibrant exercise space.

Equipped with just a few basic tools, she began exploring a variety of workouts, from heart-pumping cardio routines to muscle-building strength training exercises. Day by day, she grew stronger, more energized, and happier.

As Emily's body transformed, so did her outlook on life. She realized that getting fit at home was not only a practical solution but also a transformative experience that touched every aspect of her being. She became passionate about sharing her newfound knowledge and empowering others to embark on their home fitness journeys.

And so, dear reader, it is with great pleasure that we present to you "Get Fit at Home." This comprehensive guidebook is designed to be your companion, your cheerleader, and your source of knowledge as you embark on your path to a healthier and fitter lifestyle. Whether you're a busy professional, a stay-at-home parent, or simply someone who prefers the privacy and convenience of home workouts, this book is here to guide you every step of the way.

Within these pages, you will find a treasure trove of information, practical tips, and expert advice on how to create an effective home workout routine, regardless of your fitness level or available resources. From understanding the benefits of home fitness to setting goals, creating a workout space, and incorporating a variety of exercises into your routine, we leave no stone unturned.

But this book is more than just a manual of exercises. It's a holistic approach to fitness that recognizes the importance of nutrition, motivation, and mindset. We delve into the power of healthy eating habits, the art of staying motivated, and the strategies to overcome obstacles that may arise along your journey.

So, whether you're a beginner or an experienced fitness enthusiast, get ready to embark on an exciting adventure—one that will empower you to transform your life and achieve your fitness goals from the comfort of your own home. Let the pages of "Get Fit at Home" be your guide, and together, let's create a healthier, happier you.

Chapter 1: Understanding the Benefits of Home Fitness

Introduction:

In Chapter 1, we delve into the world of home fitness and explore the multitude of benefits it offers. Understanding these advantages will lay the foundation for your motivation and commitment to embark on your home fitness journey. Let's explore the numerous benefits that await you as you embrace the concept of getting fit at home.

1.1 Convenience:

One of the key benefits of home fitness is the unparalleled convenience it provides. No longer will you need to worry about commuting to the gym, battling traffic, or adhering to strict class schedules. With home fitness, you have the freedom to work out whenever it fits your schedule, right in the comfort of your own home.

Whether you prefer early morning workouts, late-night sessions, or quick exercise breaks throughout the day, the flexibility of home fitness ensures that you can seamlessly integrate it into your lifestyle.

1.2 Privacy and Comfort:

For many individuals, exercising in a public setting can be intimidating or uncomfortable. Home fitness eliminates those concerns by providing a private and comfortable environment to work out. You can exercise without judgment, self-consciousness, or the pressure of comparing yourself to others. Your living room, basement, or dedicated home gym becomes your sanctuary, fostering a sense of confidence and security as you focus on your fitness goals.

1.3 Cost-effectiveness:

Gym memberships, personal trainers, and specialized equipment can be costly. Home fitness offers a cost-effective alternative, allowing you to save money in the long run. You can invest in a few essential pieces of equipment or even rely solely on bodyweight exercises, and still achieve significant fitness progress.

By eliminating ongoing membership fees and the need for expensive gear, home fitness becomes an accessible and affordable option for individuals of all budgets.

1.4 Time Efficiency:

Time is a valuable resource in our modern life with its hectic pace. Home fitness eliminates the need to allocate extra time for commuting to the gym, waiting for equipment, or attending scheduled fitness classes. With workouts designed specifically for home settings, you can maximize your time by engaging in efficient and targeted exercises that deliver results in a shorter span.

Say goodbye to wasted time and hello to a more productive and effective fitness routine.

1.5 Customization and Flexibility:

One of the greatest advantages of home fitness is the ability to customize your workouts to suit your unique preferences, needs, and fitness level. You have the freedom to select exercises that align with your goals, modify routines to accommodate any physical limitations, and progress at your own pace.

Additionally, you can easily adapt your workouts to fit changing circumstances, such as travel or busy periods, ensuring that your commitment to fitness remains unwavering.

1.6 Family and Community Engagement:

Home fitness provides an excellent opportunity for family and community engagement. You can involve your loved ones in your fitness journey, creating a supportive and motivating environment.

Whether it's exercising together, encouraging healthy habits, or simply being a positive role model, home fitness can strengthen your relationships while fostering a shared commitment to well-being.

Conclusion:

Chapter 1 has provided an in-depth exploration of the benefits of home fitness. By understanding and appreciating these advantages, you are now equipped with the knowledge and motivation to embrace home fitness as a viable and transformative approach to achieving your fitness goals.

In the subsequent chapters, we will delve deeper into the practical aspects of creating your home workout space, selecting appropriate equipment, and designing effective exercise routines that will propel you toward a healthier and fitter lifestyle.

Chapter 2: Assessing Your Fitness Level

Introduction:

In Chapter 2, we focus on the critical step of assessing your current fitness level. Understanding where you stand in terms of strength, endurance, flexibility, and overall health will enable you to tailor your home fitness journey to your specific needs and goals. This chapter provides you with valuable tools and methods to assess your fitness level accurately, guiding you toward an effective and personalized workout plan.

2.1 Importance of Fitness Assessment:

Before embarking on any fitness program, it is essential to assess your starting point. A fitness assessment helps you establish a baseline, identify areas of strength and weakness, and track your progress over time. By understanding your current fitness level, you can set realistic goals and make informed decisions about the types and intensity of exercises that will benefit you the most.

2.2 Components of Fitness Assessment:

In this section, we explore the various components of fitness assessment. These include:

2.2.1 Cardiovascular Fitness:

The ability of your heart, lungs, and blood arteries to carry oxygen-rich blood to your muscles as you exercise is referred to as cardiovascular fitness. We discuss methods such as the 1-mile walk test, the 3-minute step test, or using heart rate monitors to evaluate your cardiovascular endurance.

2.2.2 Muscular Strength and Endurance:

Muscular strength is the amount of force your muscles can exert, while muscular endurance refers to their ability to sustain repeated contractions over time. We cover assessments like the push-up test, the plank hold, or using resistance bands to gauge your upper body, lower body, and core strength.

2.2.3 Flexibility:

The range of motion around a joint is called flexibility. Assessments such as the sit-and-reach test or the shoulder flexibility test will help you evaluate your flexibility level and identify any areas that require improvement.

2.2.4 Body Composition:

Body composition refers to the proportions of fat, muscle, bone, and other tissues in your body. Assessments like body mass index (BMI), skinfold measurements, or bioelectrical impedance analysis (BIA) help you determine your body fat percentage and overall body composition.

2.3 Fitness Assessment Tools:

In this section, we introduce various tools that can assist you in conducting a comprehensive fitness assessment. These tools may include fitness tracking apps, wearable devices, or fitness assessment templates that allow you to record and monitor your progress systematically.

2.4 Seeking Professional Guidance:

While self-assessment is valuable, seeking professional guidance from a fitness trainer, exercise physiologist, or healthcare provider can provide deeper insights into your fitness level. Professionals can conduct specialized assessments and help interpret the results, enabling you to develop a more personalized and effective fitness plan.

2.5 Tracking and Reassessing Your Fitness Level:

Once you have assessed your fitness level, it is crucial to track your progress regularly. We discuss the importance of tracking your workouts, measuring key indicators, and periodically reassessing your fitness level to gauge improvements and make necessary adjustments to your home fitness routine.

Conclusion:

Chapter 2 has highlighted the significance of assessing your fitness level before embarking on your home fitness journey. By evaluating your cardiovascular fitness, muscular strength and endurance, flexibility, and body composition, you gain a comprehensive understanding of your starting point. With this knowledge, you can set realistic goals, design personalized workout plans, and track your progress effectively. In Chapter 3, we will delve into goal setting and creating a plan that aligns with your assessed fitness level, propelling you toward success in your home fitness endeavors.

Chapter 3: Setting Goals and Creating a Plan

Introduction:

In Chapter 3, we dive into the vital process of setting goals and creating a comprehensive plan for your home fitness journey. Goal setting provides direction, motivation, and a sense of purpose, while a well-designed plan ensures that you stay organized and focused on your objectives. This chapter will guide you through the process of setting realistic and meaningful goals, and help you create a tailored plan that maximizes your chances of success.

3.1 Importance of Goal Setting:

Setting clear and specific goals is crucial for your home fitness journey. Goals provide a roadmap, allowing you to measure progress, stay motivated, and overcome obstacles along the way.

By establishing meaningful objectives, you can transform your vision into actionable steps that lead to tangible results.

3.2 Types of Goals:

We explore different types of goals that you can consider when setting your home fitness objectives:

3.2.1 Outcome Goals:

Outcome goals focus on the result you desire to achieve. For example, completing a specific number of push-ups, running a certain distance, or losing a certain amount of weight. Outcome goals provide a tangible target to strive for and give you a sense of accomplishment when achieved.

3.2.2 Performance Goals:

Performance goals concentrate on improving specific aspects of your fitness. These goals focus on measurable improvements in your performance, such as increasing your running speed, lifting heavier weights, or improving your flexibility. Performance goals help you monitor progress and highlight areas for improvement.

3.2.3 Process Goals:

Process goals revolve around the actions and behaviors you need to take to achieve your desired outcomes. These goals focus on consistent and sustainable habits, such as exercising a certain number of times per week, eating a balanced diet, or practicing mindfulness. Process goals provide the foundation for long-term success and help you develop positive lifestyle changes.

3.3 SMART Goal Framework:

The SMART goal framework is a valuable tool for setting goals that are specific, measurable, achievable, relevant, and time-bound. We explore each component of the SMART framework and guide you in applying it to your home fitness goals, ensuring they are well-defined and realistic.

3.4 Creating Your Fitness Plan:

Once you have established your goals, it's time to create a well-structured fitness plan.

We guide you through the process of designing a plan that aligns with your goals, preferences, and available resources. Key considerations include:

3.4.1 Exercise Selection:

Selecting exercises that align with your goals, preferences, and fitness level is essential. We provide guidance on choosing cardiovascular exercises, strength training exercises, flexibility routines, and any other modalities that suit your needs.

3.4.2 Workout Schedule:

Creating a workout schedule helps you establish a routine and ensures consistency in your training. We discuss factors to consider when designing your schedule, such as time availability, balancing different types of exercises, and incorporating rest days for recovery.

3.4.3 Progression and Periodization:

To continue making progress, it's important to incorporate progression and periodization into your plan. We explain how to gradually increase the intensity, duration, or complexity of your workouts over time.

Additionally, we discuss the concept of periodization, which involves dividing your training into distinct phases to optimize results and prevent plateaus.

3.4.4 Tracking and Accountability:

Tracking your workouts and progress is crucial for staying accountable and motivated. We explore various tracking methods, such as fitness apps, journals, or wearable devices, and discuss how tracking can help you monitor your achievements, identify patterns, and make adjustments to your plan as needed.

Conclusion:

Chapter 3 has emphasized the importance of setting goals and creating a comprehensive plan for your home fitness journey. By setting realistic and meaningful goals using the SMART framework, and designing a well-structured fitness plan that aligns with your goals and preferences, you lay a strong foundation for success. In Chapter 4, we will delve into the practical aspects of creating your home workout space, ensuring that you have an environment conducive to achieving your fitness goals.

Chapter 4: Creating Your Home Workout Space

Introduction:

In Chapter 4, we shift our focus to creating a dedicated and inspiring home workout space. Designing a well-equipped and functional area within your home will provide the necessary environment for you to engage in effective workouts, stay motivated, and fully embrace your home fitness journey. This chapter will guide you through the process of creating an ideal home workout space that suits your needs and maximizes your fitness potential.

4.1 Assessing Available Space:

The first step in creating your home workout space is to assess the available space within your home. Whether you have a spare room, a corner in your living room, or even just a small area in your bedroom, it's important to evaluate the dimensions, layout, and limitations of the space you intend to utilize.

4.2 Clearing and Organizing the Space:

To create an inviting and functional workout space, it's crucial to declutter and organize the area. We provide tips on removing unnecessary items, optimizing storage solutions, and ensuring that the space is clean and free from distractions. A clutter-free environment promotes focus and allows you to move freely during your workouts.

4.3 Lighting and Ventilation:

Proper lighting and ventilation are essential for a comfortable and energizing workout environment. We discuss the importance of natural and artificial lighting, as well as strategies to enhance the brightness and ambiance of your workout space. Additionally, we explore ventilation options to ensure proper airflow and maintain a comfortable temperature during exercise.

4.4 Flooring and Safety Considerations:

The type of flooring in your home workout space plays a crucial role in providing stability, cushioning, and shock absorption. We discuss various flooring options, such as rubber mats, foam tiles, or hardwood floors, and guide you in selecting the most appropriate choice for your specific needs. Safety considerations, such as securing loose cables, adding safety mirrors, or installing handrails, are also addressed to minimize the risk of accidents.

4.5 Essential Equipment:

In this section, we explore the essential equipment needed to equip your home workout space. Depending on your fitness goals and preferences, we discuss versatile and compact options, such as resistance bands, dumbbells, stability balls, jump ropes, or exercise mats. We emphasize the importance of selecting equipment that aligns with your workout routines and available space.

4.6 Incorporating Inspirational Elements:

To create a motivating and inspiring workout space, it's essential to incorporate elements that resonate with your fitness journey. We explore ideas for decorating the area, such as hanging motivational quotes, displaying vision boards, or incorporating plants for a touch of nature. Personalizing your space can enhance your mood, motivation, and overall enjoyment of your home workouts.

4.7 Music and Entertainment:

Music and entertainment can play a significant role in keeping you engaged and motivated during your workouts. We provide suggestions for incorporating sound systems, speakers, or portable devices to play energizing music, podcasts, or workout videos. Tailoring your workout environment to include enjoyable audio experiences can elevate your home fitness sessions.

4.8 Privacy and Distractions:

Maintaining privacy and minimizing distractions within your home workout space are important considerations for maintaining focus and maximizing productivity. We discuss strategies for creating boundaries, such as communicating with family members, setting schedules, or using room dividers, to ensure uninterrupted workout sessions.

Conclusion:

Chapter 4 has guided you on creating your home workout space—a dedicated environment that supports your fitness journey. By assessing available space, organizing and optimizing the area, selecting essential equipment, and incorporating personalized and motivational elements, you create a space that inspires and facilitates effective workouts. In Chapter 5, we delve into the essential equipment for home fitness, providing detailed information on various types of equipment and their applications in your workouts.

Chapter 5: Essential Equipment for Home Fitness

Introduction:

In Chapter 5, we explore the essential equipment needed to create an effective home fitness setup. Whether you have ample space or limited room, selecting the right equipment will enhance the variety and effectiveness of your workouts. This chapter will guide you through a comprehensive list of essential equipment options, providing insight into their uses, benefits, and considerations for incorporating them into your home fitness routine.

5.1 Importance of Essential Equipment:

Having the right equipment is crucial for maximizing the effectiveness and variety of your home workouts. These tools provide resistance, support, and assistance, enabling you to target different muscle groups, increase intensity, and achieve a well-rounded fitness program. By investing in essential equipment, you expand your exercise options and create a dynamic and challenging home workout experience.

5.2 Cardiovascular Equipment:

Exercises for the heart and lungs are an essential part of any fitness regimen. We explore essential cardio equipment options suitable for home fitness, including:

5.2.1 Treadmill: A treadmill provides a versatile option for walking, jogging, or running, allowing you to control speed and incline for effective cardiovascular workouts.

5.2.2 Stationary Bike: A stationary bike offers a low-impact cardiovascular workout that is gentle on the joints. Options include upright bikes or recumbent bikes, each providing different levels of comfort and support.

5.2.3 Elliptical Trainer: An elliptical trainer provides a low-impact, full-body workout that engages both the upper and lower body, making it an excellent choice for cardiovascular conditioning.

5.2.4 Jump Rope: A simple and affordable piece of equipment, a jump rope offers a portable and effective option for cardiovascular exercise, improving coordination, agility, and endurance.

5.3 Strength Training Equipment:

Strength training is essential for building and toning muscles, improving bone density, and increasing overall strength. We explore various options for strength training equipment suitable for home fitness, including:

5.3.1 Dumbbells: Dumbbells are versatile and allow for a wide range of exercises targeting different muscle groups. They come in various weights and can be adjustable or fixed.

5.3.2 Resistance Bands: Resistance bands offer a portable and cost-effective option for strength training. They provide varying levels of resistance and can be used for a variety of exercises, targeting different muscle groups.

5.3.3 Kettlebells: Kettlebells provide a dynamic and functional strength training option, engaging multiple muscle groups simultaneously. They come in different weights and offer versatility for various exercises.

5.3.4 Adjustable Weight Bench: An adjustable weight bench provides support and stability for a range of exercises, such as chest presses, shoulder presses, and step-ups.

5.4 Flexibility and Mobility Equipment:

Flexibility and mobility exercises are essential for maintaining joint health, improving posture, and preventing injuries. We explore equipment options that can aid in stretching and improving flexibility, including:

5.4.1 Yoga Mat: A yoga mat provides a comfortable and non-slip surface for various stretching exercises, yoga poses, or bodyweight exercises.

5.4.2 Foam Roller: A foam roller is used for self-myofascial release, helping to relieve muscle tension, improve flexibility, and enhance recovery.

5.4.3 Stretching Strap: A stretching strap assists in improving flexibility and range of motion by providing support during stretching exercises.

5.5 Additional Equipment Options:

In this section, we discuss additional equipment options that can enhance your home fitness routine:

5.5.1 Stability Ball: A stability ball, also known as an exercise ball, is versatile and can be used for core exercises, stability exercises, and improving balance.

5.5.2 Pull-Up Bar: A pull-up bar allows for upper body strengthening exercises, such as pull-ups and chin-ups, and can be mounted on a doorway or secured to a wall.

5.5.3 Suspension Trainer: A suspension trainer utilizes bodyweight exercises, providing a full-body workout that improves strength, stability, and flexibility.

5.5.4 Fitness Step Platform: A fitness step platform offers versatility for aerobic exercises, step-ups, and other lower body strengthening exercises.

Conclusion:

Chapter 5 has explored the essential equipment for home fitness, covering options for cardiovascular exercise, strength training, flexibility, and mobility. By incorporating these equipment choices into your home workout space, you can elevate the effectiveness and variety of your workouts, ensuring a well-rounded and challenging fitness program. In Chapter 6, we delve into cardiovascular exercises that can be performed at home, guiding how to improve cardiovascular fitness and enhance your overall health.

Chapter 6: Cardiovascular Exercises at Home

Introduction:

In Chapter 6, we shift our focus to cardiovascular exercises that can be performed at home. Cardiovascular exercise, also known as aerobic exercise, is essential for improving cardiovascular health, increasing endurance, burning calories, and boosting overall fitness. This chapter will guide you through a variety of effective cardiovascular exercises that you can incorporate into your home fitness routine, ensuring a well-rounded and heart-pumping workout experience.

6.1 Importance of Cardiovascular Exercise:

Cardiovascular exercise offers numerous health benefits and plays a crucial role in maintaining overall fitness.

It strengthens the heart, improves lung capacity, enhances circulation, and helps manage weight. Engaging in regular cardiovascular exercise boosts energy levels, reduces the risk of chronic diseases, and improves mental well-being. Incorporating cardiovascular exercises into your home fitness routine will enhance your overall health and fitness.

6.2 Types of Cardiovascular Exercises:

In this section, we explore a range of cardiovascular exercises that can be performed at home, providing options suitable for different fitness levels and preferences:

6.2.1 Jumping Jacks: Jumping jacks are a simple yet effective full-body exercise that elevates the heart rate, improves coordination, and engages multiple muscle groups.

6.2.2 High Knees: High knees involve running in place while lifting your knees as high as possible. This exercise elevates the heart rate, engages the core, and strengthens the lower body.

6.2.3 Burpees: Burpees are a challenging and dynamic exercise that combines squats, push-ups, and jumps. They provide a total-body workout, increasing cardiovascular endurance and building strength.

6.2.4 Mountain Climbers: Mountain climbers target the core, shoulders, and legs while elevating the heart rate. They simulate climbing movements and help improve coordination and agility.

6.2.5 Jump Rope: Jumping rope is a classic cardiovascular exercise that can be done with minimal space and equipment. It improves coordination, cardiovascular endurance, and lower body strength.

6.2.6 Running or Jogging in Place: Running or jogging in place is a convenient cardiovascular exercise that requires minimal space. It effectively elevates the heart rate, burns calories, and improves endurance.

6.2.7 High-Intensity Interval Training (HIIT): HIIT involves switching between short rest periods and high-intensity training sessions. It can include exercises such as squat jumps, burpees, or high knees, providing an efficient and intense cardiovascular workout.

6.2.8 Dancing: Dancing is a fun and engaging way to get your heart rate up and improve cardiovascular fitness. You can follow dance workout videos or move to your favorite tunes.

6.3 Designing a Cardiovascular Workout:

Creating a well-structured cardiovascular workout is essential for maximizing the benefits of these exercises. We guide you in designing a cardiovascular workout routine that suits your fitness level, goals, and time availability. Considerations include:

6.3.1 Warm-up: Always begin your cardiovascular workout with a warm-up to prepare your body for exercise. This may involve dynamic stretches, marching in place, or light cardio movements.

6.3.2 Work-to-Rest Ratio: Determine the duration and intensity of each cardiovascular exercise, as well as the rest periods in between. You can tailor these ratios based on your fitness level and goals.

6.3.3 Progression: As you improve your cardiovascular fitness, gradually increase the duration, intensity, or complexity of your exercises to continue challenging your body and achieving progress.

6.3.4 Cool-down: End your cardiovascular workout with a cool-down period to gradually bring your heart rate down and stretch your muscles. This promotes recovery and reduces the risk of muscle soreness.

6.4 Incorporating Cardiovascular Exercise Into Your Routine:

To ensure consistency and adherence, it's important to find ways to incorporate cardiovascular exercise into your daily routine. We discuss strategies such as scheduling dedicated cardio sessions, integrating cardio intervals into strength training workouts, or engaging in active hobbies that elevate your heart rate.

Conclusion:

Chapter 6 has explored various cardiovascular exercises that can be performed at home, providing options to improve cardiovascular fitness and boost overall health. By incorporating these exercises into your home fitness routine and designing a well-structured cardiovascular workout, you can elevate your endurance, burn calories, and enhance your overall fitness level. In Chapter 7, we delve into strength training exercises that can be done at home, focusing on building strength, toning muscles, and improving functional fitness.

Chapter 7: Strength Training at Home

Introduction:

In Chapter 7, we delve into the world of strength training exercises that can be done at home. Strength training is crucial for building and toning muscles, increasing bone density, improving posture, and enhancing overall strength and functionality. This chapter will guide you through a variety of effective strength training exercises that can be incorporated into your home fitness routine, ensuring a well-rounded and empowering workout experience.

7.1 Importance of Strength Training:

Beyond merely enhancing muscle growth, strength training has many other advantages. It improves bone health, boosts metabolism, enhances joint stability, and promotes functional fitness.

Engaging in regular strength training exercises at home will help you achieve a balanced and strong physique while improving your overall health and physical performance.

7.2 Bodyweight Exercises:

Bodyweight exercises are an excellent starting point for strength training at home, as they require no equipment and can be performed anywhere. We explore a range of bodyweight exercises that target different muscle groups, including:

7.2.1 Push-Ups: Push-ups primarily target the chest, shoulders, and triceps, but also engage the core and back muscles.

7.2.2 Squats: Squats are a compound exercise that targets the lower body, including the quadriceps, hamstrings, and glutes.

7.2.3 Lunges: Lunges work the lower body muscles, including the quadriceps, hamstrings, glutes, and calves.

7.2.4 Plank: Planks engage the core muscles, including the abdominals, back, and shoulders, promoting stability and strength.

7.2.5 Glute Bridges: Glute bridges activate the glute muscles, helping to strengthen the hips, lower back, and hamstrings.

7.2.6 Superman Pose: The Superman pose targets the muscles of the lower back, glutes, and hamstrings, promoting a strong posterior chain.

7.3 Resistance Band Exercises:

Resistance bands are a versatile and affordable tool for strength training at home. They provide resistance throughout the range of motion, effectively challenging your muscles. We explore a variety of resistance band exercises that target different muscle groups, including:

7.3.1 Bicep Curls: Bicep curls with resistance bands target the bicep muscles, helping to build strength and tone the arms.

7.3.2 Standing Rows: Standing rows engage the back muscles, including the rhomboids, upper back, and rear deltoids.

7.3.3 Glute Kickbacks: Glute kickbacks with resistance bands isolate and activate the glute muscles, helping to sculpt and strengthen the buttocks.

7.3.4 Shoulder Press: The shoulder press with resistance bands targets the shoulder muscles, including the deltoids and trapezius.

7.3.5 Leg Press: The leg press exercise using resistance bands targets the quadriceps, hamstrings, and glutes, providing a challenging lower-body workout.

7.4 Dumbbell Exercises:

Dumbbells are a versatile and effective tool for strength training at home, allowing for a wide range of exercises. We explore a variety of dumbbell exercises that target different muscle groups, including:

7.4.1 Dumbbell Chest Press: The dumbbell chest press targets the chest muscles, triceps, and shoulders, helping to build upper body strength.

7.4.2 Dumbbell Rows: Dumbbell rows engage the back muscles, including the lats, rhomboids, and rear deltoids.

7.4.3 Dumbbell Lunges: Dumbbell lunges add resistance to the lower body exercise, targeting the quadriceps, hamstrings, and glutes.

7.4.4 Dumbbell Shoulder Press: The dumbbell shoulder press targets the deltoid muscles, promoting shoulder strength and stability.

7.4.5 Dumbbell Deadlifts: Dumbbell deadlifts engage the posterior chain muscles, including the glutes, hamstrings, and lower back.

7.5 Designing a Strength Training Routine:

Designing a well-structured strength training routine is essential for maximizing the benefits of these exercises.

We guide you in designing a routine that suits your fitness level, goals, and time availability. Considerations include:

7.5.1 Exercise Selection: Choose a variety of exercises that target different muscle groups to ensure a well-rounded workout.

7.5.2 Sets and Repetitions: Determine the number of sets and repetitions that best suit your fitness level and goals. Set an ambitious but reasonable workload goal.

7.5.3 Rest Periods: Allow sufficient rest between sets to promote recovery and optimize performance.

7.5.4 Progression: Gradually increase the weight, repetitions, or difficulty of your exercises over time to continue challenging your muscles and making progress.

Conclusion:

Chapter 7 has explored a variety of strength training exercises that can be done at home, ranging from bodyweight exercises to resistance bands and dumbbell exercises. By incorporating these exercises into your home fitness routine and designing a well-structured strength training routine, you can build strength, tone muscles, and improve your overall functional fitness. In Chapter 8, we delve into flexibility and stretching exercises, focusing on improving joint mobility, preventing injuries, and enhancing overall flexibility.

Chapter 8: Flexibility and Stretching Exercises

Introduction:

In Chapter 8, we explore the importance of flexibility and stretching exercises as a vital component of your home fitness routine. Flexibility exercises help improve joint mobility, increase range of motion, prevent injuries, and enhance overall physical performance. This chapter will guide you through a variety of effective stretching exercises that can be incorporated into your home fitness routine, ensuring a well-rounded and balanced approach to your fitness journey.

8.1 Importance of Flexibility and Stretching:

Flexibility plays a crucial role in maintaining overall physical health and fitness. By incorporating flexibility and stretching exercises into your home fitness routine, you can improve posture, reduce muscle tension, enhance athletic performance, and prevent injuries. Flexibility exercises also promote relaxation and improve circulation, contributing to overall well-being.

8.2 Dynamic Stretching:

Dynamic stretching involves moving your muscles and joints through a full range of motion, mimicking the movements of your workout or activity. These stretches help warm up the body, increase blood flow to the muscles, and prepare them for activity. We explore a variety of dynamic stretching exercises, including:

8.2.1 Arm Circles: Arm circles warm up the shoulders and upper body, promoting flexibility and range of motion.

8.2.2 Leg Swings: Leg swings target the hip flexors, hamstrings, and glutes, improving flexibility and mobility in the lower body.

8.2.3 Torso Twists: Torso twists engage the core muscles and promote spinal mobility, enhancing overall flexibility.

8.2.4 Walking Lunges: Walking lunges combine stretching with lower body strengthening, targeting the quadriceps, hamstrings, and hip flexors.

8.2.5 Shoulder Circles: Shoulder circles help warm up and mobilize the shoulder joints, improving flexibility and reducing the risk of injury.

8.3 Static Stretching:

Static stretching involves holding a stretch position for a prolonged period, allowing the muscles to lengthen and relax. These stretches are typically done after a workout or physical activity to cool down and improve flexibility. We explore a variety of static stretching exercises, including:

8.3.1 Hamstring Stretch: The hamstring stretch targets the back of the thighs, improving flexibility and reducing muscle tightness.

8.3.2 Quadriceps Stretch: The quadriceps stretch targets the front of the thighs, promoting flexibility and relieving muscle tension.

8.3.3 Chest Stretch: The chest stretch helps counteract the effects of prolonged sitting and hunching, improving posture and chest flexibility.

8.3.4 Hip Flexor Stretch: The hip flexor stretch targets the muscles at the front of the hips, promoting flexibility and reducing hip tightness.

8.3.5 Tricep Stretch: The tricep stretch targets the muscles at the back of the upper arms, enhancing flexibility and reducing muscle tightness.

8.4 Yoga and Pilates:

For increasing flexibility, strength, and body awareness, try yoga or pilates. We discuss the benefits of incorporating yoga and Pilates exercises into your home fitness routine, guiding specific poses and exercises that promote flexibility and enhance overall well-being.

8.5 Incorporating Flexibility Exercises:

To ensure consistency and adherence, it's important to find ways to incorporate flexibility exercises into your daily routine. We discuss strategies such as dedicating specific time for stretching, incorporating stretches as part of your warm-up and cool-down routines, and combining flexibility exercises with other activities, such as watching TV or listening to music.

8.6 Guidelines for Safe Stretching:

Stretching should be done safely to avoid injury and maximize its benefits. We provide guidelines for safe stretching, including:

8.6.1 Warm-Up: Always warm up your muscles before stretching by performing light cardio exercises or dynamic stretching.

8.6.2 Gentle and Controlled Movements: Move into each stretch slowly and avoid bouncing or jerking movements, which can strain the muscles.

8.6.3 Comfortable Stretch: Stretch to the point of mild tension or discomfort, but never to the point of pain. Pay attention to your body's signals and be mindful of its limitations.

8.6.4 Breathe and Relax: Take deep, relaxed breaths while stretching to encourage relaxation and promote a deeper stretch.

Conclusion:

Chapter 8 has explored the importance of flexibility and stretching exercises as an integral part of your home fitness routine. By incorporating dynamic and static stretching exercises, exploring yoga and Pilates practices, and following guidelines for safe stretching, you can improve flexibility, prevent injuries, and enhance overall physical performance. In Chapter 9, we will discuss the role of nutrition in supporting your home fitness journey, providing guidance on healthy eating habits, and fueling your workouts effectively.

Chapter 9: Incorporating HIIT (High-Intensity Interval Training)

Introduction:

In Chapter 9, we explore the concept of High-Intensity Interval Training (HIIT) and its benefits for your home fitness routine. HIIT involves short bursts of intense exercise followed by brief recovery periods, offering an efficient and effective way to improve cardiovascular fitness, burn calories, and boost overall athletic performance. This chapter will guide you through incorporating HIIT into your home workouts, providing insight into its principles, sample workouts, and considerations for optimal results.

9.1 Understanding HIIT:

High-Intensity Interval Training involves alternating between high-intensity exercise intervals and short periods of active recovery or rest.

This approach challenges both aerobic and anaerobic energy systems, resulting in increased calorie burn and improved cardiovascular fitness. HIIT sessions are typically shorter in duration compared to steady-state cardio workouts, making them ideal for those with limited time or looking for a time-efficient exercise solution.

9.2 Benefits of HIIT:

Incorporating HIIT into your home fitness routine offers several benefits:

9.2.1 Improved Cardiovascular Fitness: HIIT elevates your heart rate, pushing your cardiovascular system to adapt and become more efficient at delivering oxygen to working muscles.

9.2.2 Increased Caloric Expenditure: The intense nature of HIIT workouts leads to a higher post-workout calorie burn, known as excess post-exercise oxygen consumption (EPOC). This means you continue to burn calories even after the workout is finished.

9.2.3 Time Efficiency: HIIT workouts can be completed in a shorter amount of time compared to traditional cardio sessions, making them a convenient option for those with busy schedules.

9.2.4 Muscle Preservation: HIIT workouts help preserve muscle mass while promoting fat loss, as they are designed to retain muscle and primarily target fat stores.

9.2.5 Versatility: HIIT can be adapted to various exercises, such as running, cycling, bodyweight exercises, or even using equipment like kettlebells or dumbbells. This versatility allows for a wide range of workout options based on your preferences and available resources.

9.3 Principles of HIIT:

To structure an effective HIIT workout, it's essential to understand and apply certain principles:

9.3.1 Work-to-Rest Ratio: HIIT involves alternating periods of high-intensity exercise with recovery or rest periods.

The work-to-rest ratio can vary depending on fitness level and goals. Common ratios include 1:1 (equal work and rest), 2:1 (twice as long rest as work), or even shorter rest periods for more advanced individuals.

9.3.2 Intensity: The high-intensity intervals of HIIT should be challenging, pushing you to your maximum effort. This intensity is subjective and can be adjusted based on your fitness level and capabilities.

9.3.3 Exercise Selection: Choose exercises that engage large muscle groups and allow for intense efforts, such as sprinting, squat jumps, burpees, or kettlebell swings. This helps maximize calorie burn and overall impact.

9.3.4 Progression: As with any exercise program, it's important to progressively increase the intensity or duration of HIIT workouts over time to continue challenging your body and promoting improvement.

9.4 Sample HIIT Workouts:

In this section, we provide sample HIIT workouts that you can incorporate into your home fitness routine.

These workouts can be modified based on your fitness level and preferences. It's important to warm up adequately before starting any HIIT session.

9.4.1 Tabata: Tabata is a popular HIIT protocol that involves 20 seconds of intense exercise followed by 10 seconds of rest, repeated for a total of four minutes. This pattern can be repeated multiple times with different exercises.

9.4.2 30-Second Intervals: Perform exercises at a high intensity for 30 seconds, followed by 30 seconds of active recovery. Repeat this pattern for a set number of rounds or desired duration.

9.4.3 Pyramid: Start with a short burst of high-intensity exercise, such as 10 seconds, followed by a brief rest period. Gradually increase the work duration in increments (e.g., 20 seconds, 30 seconds, 40 seconds), followed by the same duration of rest. Once you reach the peak duration, gradually decrease the work duration back down the pyramid.

9.5 Considerations for Optimal Results:

To maximize the benefits of incorporating HIIT into your home fitness routine, consider the following:

9.5.1 Proper Form: Focus on maintaining proper form throughout each exercise to minimize the risk of injury and ensure optimal effectiveness.

9.5.2 Recovery: Allow adequate recovery between HIIT sessions to allow for muscle repair and adaptation. Aim for at least one or two days of rest or lower-intensity activities per week.

9.5.3 Listen to Your Body: HIIT can be demanding, so pay attention to your body's signals and adjust the intensity or rest periods as needed. It's important to challenge yourself but also know your limits.

9.5.4 Progress Gradually: Start with shorter intervals and lower intensities if you're new to HIIT, gradually increasing the duration or intensity over time as you become more comfortable and conditioned.

Conclusion:

Chapter 9 has introduced the concept of High-Intensity Interval Training (HIIT) and its benefits for your home fitness routine. By incorporating HIIT workouts into your exercise regimen, you can improve cardiovascular fitness, increase calorie burn, and enhance overall athletic performance. Understanding the principles of HIIT, structuring sample workouts, and considering key factors for optimal results will allow you to reap the rewards of this efficient and effective training method. In Chapter 10, we will explore the importance of recovery and rest in your home fitness journey, highlighting strategies to optimize recovery and promote overall well-being.

Chapter 10: Bodyweight Exercises for Full-Body Workouts

Introduction:

In Chapter 10, we explore the power of bodyweight exercises for achieving full-body workouts at home. Bodyweight exercises utilize your own body as resistance, requiring no additional equipment, making them accessible and convenient for all fitness levels. This chapter will guide you through a variety of effective bodyweight exercises that target different muscle groups, helping you develop strength, endurance, and overall fitness without the need for specialized equipment.

10.1 Benefits of Bodyweight Exercises:

Incorporating bodyweight exercises into your home fitness routine offers several benefits:

10.1.1 Convenience and Accessibility: Bodyweight exercises can be performed anywhere, requiring minimal space and no equipment. This makes them highly accessible and convenient for home workouts.

10.1.2 Full-Body Engagement: Bodyweight exercises often engage multiple muscle groups simultaneously, providing a well-rounded workout that improves overall strength and stability.

10.1.3 Functional Strength: Bodyweight exercises mimic natural movements and develop functional strength, enhancing your ability to perform daily activities and sports with efficiency and reduced risk of injury.

10.1.4 Body Control and Coordination: Performing bodyweight exercises requires control and coordination, improving your overall body awareness and movement proficiency.

10.1.5 Scalability: Bodyweight exercises can be modified to suit different fitness levels by adjusting the range of motion, intensity, or complexity of the movements.

10.2 Upper Body Exercises:

We explore a variety of bodyweight exercises that target the upper body muscles, including:

10.2.1 Push-Ups: Push-ups engage the chest, shoulders, triceps, and core muscles, developing upper body strength and stability.

10.2.2 Dips: Dips primarily target the triceps, chest, and shoulders, helping to develop arm and upper body strength.

10.2.3 Plank Variations: Planks strengthen the core, including the abdominals, back, and shoulders, promoting stability and improved posture.

10.2.4 Pike Push-Ups: Pike push-ups target the shoulders, upper chest, and triceps, providing a challenging exercise for upper body strength.

10.3 Lower Body Exercises:

We explore a variety of bodyweight exercises that target the lower body muscles, including:

10.3.1 Squats: Squats engage the quadriceps, hamstrings, and glutes, developing lower body strength and stability.

10.3.2 Lunges: Lunges work the quadriceps, hamstrings, glutes, and calves, promoting leg strength and balance.

10.3.3 Glute Bridges: Glute bridges target the glute muscles, helping to strengthen the hips, lower back, and hamstrings.

10.3.4 Step-Ups: Step-ups engage the lower body muscles, including the quadriceps, hamstrings, and glutes, providing a functional exercise for leg strength and balance.

10.4 Core Exercises:

We explore a variety of bodyweight exercises that target the core muscles, including:

10.4.1 Plank: Planks engage the entire core, including the abdominals, back, and shoulders, promoting stability and improved posture.

10.4.2 Russian Twists: Russian twists target the obliques and core muscles, improving rotational strength and stability.

10.4.3 Bicycle Crunches: Bicycle crunches engage the abdominal muscles, including the rectus abdominis and obliques, promoting core strength and definition.

10.4.4 Mountain Climbers: Mountain climbers work the core, shoulders, and legs, providing a dynamic exercise for overall core stability and cardiovascular fitness.

10.5 Full-Body Exercises:

We explore a variety of bodyweight exercises that engage multiple muscle groups and provide full-body benefits, including:

10.5.1 Burpees: Burpees combine squat jumps, push-ups, and jumps, providing a challenging full-body exercise that builds strength and cardiovascular fitness.

10.5.2 Plank-to-Push-Up: Plank-to-push-up transitions engage the core, upper body, and lower body, promoting overall strength and stability.

10.5.3 Inchworms: Inchworms target the core, shoulders, and hamstrings, improving flexibility, strength, and body control.

10.5.4 Mountain Climbers: Mountain climbers engage the core, shoulders, and legs, providing a dynamic exercise for overall strength and cardiovascular fitness.

10.6 Creating a Full-Body Workout:

To design an effective full-body workout using bodyweight exercises, consider the following:

10.6.1 Exercise Selection: Choose a variety of exercises that target different muscle groups to ensure a balanced and challenging workout.

10.6.2 Repetitions and Sets: Determine the number of repetitions and sets that suit your fitness level and goals. Set an ambitious but reasonable workload goal.

10.6.3 Rest Periods: Allow sufficient rest between sets to promote recovery and optimize performance. Rest periods can vary depending on the intensity of the exercises and your fitness level.

10.6.4 Progression: As with any exercise program, gradually increase the difficulty or intensity of the exercises over time to continue challenging your body and promoting improvement.

Conclusion:

Chapter 10 has explored the power of bodyweight exercises for achieving full-body workouts at home. By incorporating upper-body, lower-body, core, and full-body exercises into your home fitness routine, you can develop strength, endurance, and overall fitness without the need for specialized equipment. Understanding the benefits of bodyweight exercises, selecting appropriate exercises, and designing a well-rounded full-body workout will help you maximize the effectiveness of your home workouts

Chapter 11: Yoga and Pilates for Strength and Balance

Introduction:

In Chapter 11, we delve into the world of Yoga and Pilates as powerful practices for developing strength, flexibility, and balance in your home fitness routine. Both Yoga and Pilates focus on mindful movement, proper alignment, and breath control, offering a holistic approach to physical fitness and mental well-being. This chapter will guide you through various Yoga and Pilates exercises and their benefits, helping you enhance strength, improve posture, and cultivate balance in your body and mind.

11.1 Understanding Yoga:

Yoga is an ancient practice that combines physical postures (asanas), breathing techniques (pranayama), and meditation to promote overall well-being. The practice of Yoga offers a range of benefits, including:

11.1.1 Increased Flexibility: Yoga poses help improve flexibility by stretching and elongating the muscles, ligaments, and tendons.

11.1.2 Strength Development: Yoga poses require engaging various muscle groups, promoting strength and stability throughout the body.

11.1.3 Improved Posture: Practicing Yoga helps align the spine and improve posture, reducing strain on the joints and supporting optimal body mechanics.

11.1.4 Stress Reduction: Yoga incorporates breath control and meditation, promoting relaxation and reducing stress levels.

11.1.5 Mind-Body Connection: Yoga encourages mindfulness and awareness of the body, fostering a deeper connection between the mind and body.

11.2 Yoga Poses for Strength and Flexibility:

We explore a variety of Yoga poses that can be practiced at home, targeting strength, flexibility, and balance, including:

11.2.1 Downward Facing Dog (Adho Mukha Svanasana): Downward Facing Dog stretches and strengthens the entire body, particularly the shoulders, hamstrings, and calves.

11.2.2 Warrior II (Virabhadrasana II): Warrior II enhances balance and stability while strengthening the legs and core.

11.2.3 Tree Pose (Vrikshasana): Tree Pose improves balance and strengthens the legs, while also promoting focus and concentration.

11.2.4 Plank Pose (Phalakasana): Plank Pose engages the core, arms, and legs, building strength and stability throughout the body.

11.2.5 Bridge Pose (Setu Bandhasana): Bridge Pose strengthens the glutes, hamstrings, and back muscles, promoting spinal flexibility and stability.

11.3 Understanding Pilates:

Pilates is a low-impact exercise method that focuses on core strength, alignment, and controlled movements. Pilates offers numerous benefits, including:

11.3.1 Core Strength: Pilates exercises primarily target the deep core muscles, including the abdominals, back, and pelvic floor, promoting a strong and stable core.

11.3.2 Improved Posture: Pilates emphasizes proper alignment and spinal awareness, leading to improved posture and reduced risk of musculoskeletal imbalances.

11.3.3 Increased Flexibility: Pilates exercises incorporate dynamic stretching and lengthening movements, improving overall flexibility and range of motion.

11.3.4 Balanced Muscle Development: Pilates exercises promote balanced muscle development, ensuring that all muscle groups are strengthened and equally engaged.

11.3.5 Mind-Body Connection: Pilates encourages mindfulness and precise movements, fostering a deeper connection between the mind and body.

11.4 Pilates Exercises for Strength and Stability:

We explore a variety of Pilates exercises that can be performed at home, targeting strength, stability, and body awareness, including:

11.4.1 Hundred: The Hundred exercise engages the core, strengthens the abdominals, and improves overall endurance.

11.4.2 Pilates Roll-Up: The Roll-Up exercise targets the abdominals, back, and hip flexors, promoting core strength and flexibility.

11.4.3 Single Leg Circles: Single Leg Circles improve hip mobility, core stability, and leg strength.

11.4.4 Swan Dive: The Swan Dive exercise strengthens the back muscles, improves posture, and promotes spinal extension.

11.4.5 Side Plank: Side Plank targets the obliques, shoulders, and hips, enhancing core stability and lateral strength.

11.5 Incorporating Yoga and Pilates into Your Routine:

To reap the benefits of Yoga and Pilates, consider the following:

11.5.1 Frequency: Aim to incorporate Yoga and Pilates exercises into your routine at least a few times per week to experience the benefits consistently.

11.5.2 Guided Classes: Joining online Yoga or Pilates classes can provide guidance and structure, helping you learn proper technique and progress in your practice.

11.5.3 Breathing and Mindfulness: Focus on conscious breathing and mindfulness during Yoga and Pilates exercises, connecting your body, breath, and mind.

11.5.4 Modification and Progression: Modify poses or exercises as needed to suit your current fitness level and gradually progress as you build strength and flexibility.

Conclusion:

Chapter 11 has explored the benefits of incorporating Yoga and Pilates into your home fitness routine. By practicing Yoga and Pilates exercises, you can enhance strength, improve flexibility, and cultivate balance in both your body and mind. Understanding the principles of Yoga and Pilates, incorporating specific poses and exercises, and focusing on breath control and mindfulness will allow you to harness the transformative power of these practices. In Chapter 12, we will discuss the importance of recovery and rest in your home fitness journey, highlighting strategies to optimize recovery, prevent injuries, and promote overall well-being.

Chapter 12: Nutrition and Healthy Eating Habits

Introduction:

In Chapter 12, we explore the vital role of nutrition and healthy eating habits in supporting your home fitness journey. Proper nutrition provides the essential nutrients your body needs for optimal performance, muscle recovery, and overall well-being. This chapter will guide you through the fundamentals of nutrition, offering practical tips and advice for nourishing your body and achieving your fitness goals.

12.1 Understanding Nutrition:

Nutrition is the process of providing your body with the necessary nutrients, vitamins, and minerals it needs to function properly. It plays a crucial role in fueling your workouts, promoting muscle growth and repair, and maintaining overall health.

Understanding the key components of nutrition will help you make informed choices about your diet.

12.1.1 Macronutrients: Macronutrients include carbohydrates, proteins, and fats. They assist many bodily processes and give energy. Balancing macronutrients is essential for achieving optimal health and fitness.

12.1.2 Micronutrients: Micronutrients refer to vitamins and minerals that are necessary for your body's proper functioning. They are involved in processes such as energy production, immune function, and muscle repair.

12.1.3 Hydration: Proper hydration is essential for overall health and exercise performance. Water aids in controlling body temperature, moving nutrients, and removing waste.

12.2 Building a Balanced Plate:

Creating a balanced plate ensures you consume a variety of nutrients necessary for your fitness journey. Consider the following:

12.2.1 Carbohydrates: Include complex carbohydrates such as whole grains, fruits, and vegetables. They provide energy for your workouts and promote satiety.

12.2.2 Proteins: Choose lean sources of protein such as poultry, fish, legumes, and tofu. Protein supports muscle repair and growth.

12.2.3 Fats: Include healthy fats from sources like nuts, seeds, avocados, and olive oil. They provide energy and support overall health.

12.2.4 Vegetables and Fruits: Fill half of your plate with a variety of colorful vegetables and fruits. They are rich in vitamins, minerals, and fiber.

12.2.5 Portion Control: Be mindful of portion sizes to avoid overeating. To better regulate servings, use smaller dishes and bowls.

12.3 Pre-Workout Nutrition:

Fueling your body before a workout is essential for optimal performance and energy levels. Consider the following pre-workout nutrition tips:

12.3.1 Carbohydrates: Consume a small portion of easily digestible carbohydrates before your workout, such as a banana or whole grain toast. This provides readily available energy.

12.3.2 Protein: Include a small amount of protein, such as Greek yogurt or a protein shake, to support muscle repair and maintenance.

12.3.3 Timing: Eat a pre-workout meal or snack 1-2 hours before your exercise session to allow for digestion.

12.3.4 Hydration: Drink water before your workout to ensure proper hydration.

12.4 Post-Workout Nutrition:

After a workout, your body requires nutrients to replenish energy stores and support muscle recovery. Consider the following post-workout nutrition tips:

12.4.1 Carbohydrates: Consume carbohydrates to replenish glycogen stores. Choose complex carbohydrates like whole wheat bread, sweet potatoes, or brown rice.

12.4.2 Protein: Include a source of lean protein, such as chicken breast, eggs, or tofu, to support muscle repair and growth.

12.4.3 Timing: Consume a post-workout meal or snack within 30 minutes to an hour after exercise to maximize nutrient uptake.

12.4.4 Hydration: Rehydrate by drinking water or a sports drink containing electrolytes to replenish fluids lost during the workout.

12.5 Healthy Eating Habits:

Adopting healthy eating habits is essential for long-term success. Consider the following tips:

12.5.1 Meal Planning: Plan your meals ahead of time to ensure a balanced and nutritious diet. This helps avoid impulsive and unhealthy food choices.

12.5.2 Mindful Eating: Practice mindful eating by paying attention to hunger and fullness cues, savoring each bite, and avoiding distractions during meals.

12.5.3 Moderation: Enjoy a variety of foods in moderation, including occasional treats. Restrictive diets often lead to feelings of deprivation and can be difficult to sustain.

12.5.4 Listen to Your Body: Learn to recognize your body's signals of hunger and fullness. Eat only when you are hungry, and only until you are full.

12.6 Seeking Professional Guidance:

Consider speaking with a trained dietitian or nutritionist if you have certain dietary requirements or objectives. They can provide personalized guidance based on your individual needs, preferences, and fitness goals.

Conclusion:

Chapter 12 has emphasized the importance of nutrition and healthy eating habits in supporting your home fitness journey. By understanding the fundamentals of nutrition, building balanced plates, fueling properly before and after workouts, and adopting healthy eating habits, you can optimize your fitness results, support muscle recovery, and enhance overall well-being. Remember, proper nutrition is a key pillar of a sustainable and successful fitness lifestyle. In Chapter 13, we will discuss the significance of rest and recovery, highlighting strategies to optimize recovery, prevent injuries, and promote overall well-being in your home fitness routine.

Chapter 13: Staying Motivated and Overcoming Obstacles

Introduction:

In Chapter 13, we delve into the essential topic of staying motivated and overcoming obstacles in your home fitness journey. Maintaining motivation and overcoming challenges is crucial for achieving your fitness goals and sustaining a healthy lifestyle. This chapter will provide you with strategies, tips, and techniques to help you stay motivated, overcome obstacles, and continue progressing toward your desired fitness outcomes.

13.1 Setting Clear Goals:

Setting clear and specific goals is the foundation of staying motivated. Consider the following tips for goal setting:

13.1.1 Define Your Goals: Clearly define what you want to achieve, whether it's weight loss, muscle gain, improved endurance, or overall fitness.

13.1.2 Make Them Specific: Set specific and measurable goals, such as "lose 10 pounds in three months" or "run a 5K race in under 30 minutes."

13.1.3 Break It Down: Break larger goals into smaller, achievable milestones to track progress and maintain motivation.

13.1.4 Write It Down: Write your goals down and display them in a visible place to remind yourself of what you're working towards.

13.2 Finding Intrinsic Motivation:

Intrinsic motivation comes from within and is essential for long-term success. Consider the following strategies for finding and cultivating intrinsic motivation:

13.2.1 Identify Your Why: Reflect on why you want to achieve your fitness goals. Focus on the deeper reasons that resonate with your values and personal aspirations.

13.2.2 Celebrate Progress: Acknowledge and celebrate your achievements along the way, no matter how small. This will reinforce your sense of accomplishment and motivation.

13.2.3 Create a Reward System: Establish a reward system for yourself, where you reward yourself with non-food treats or activities when you reach certain milestones.

13.2.4 Find Joy in the Process: Enjoy the journey rather than solely focus on the result. Find joy in the workouts, the process of improving, and the positive changes you experience along the way.

13.3 Building a Support System:

Having a support system can significantly impact your motivation and ability to overcome obstacles. Take into account the following methods for creating a support network:

13.3.1 Share Your Goals: Share your fitness goals with supportive friends, family members, or online communities. Their encouragement and accountability can help keep you motivated.

13.3.2 Find a Workout Buddy: Partnering up with a workout buddy can provide companionship, motivation, and friendly competition, making your fitness journey more enjoyable.

13.3.3 Join Fitness Classes or Groups: Participate in fitness classes or groups, either in-person or online, where you can connect with like-minded individuals and draw inspiration from their dedication and progress.

13.3.4 Hire a Professional: Consider working with a personal trainer or fitness coach who can provide expertise, guidance, and support tailored to your needs and goals.

13.4 Overcoming Obstacles:

Obstacles are inevitable in any fitness journey, but with the right mindset and strategies, they can be overcome. Consider the following techniques for overcoming obstacles:

13.4.1 Embrace a Growth Mindset: Adopt a growth mindset that sees challenges as opportunities for growth and learning. Shift your perspective from seeing obstacles as setbacks to seeing them as stepping stones toward your goals.

13.4.2 Problem-Solving: Analyze the obstacles you encounter and brainstorm solutions. To make them more attainable, divide them into more doable, smaller steps.

13.4.3 Modify Your Approach: If a particular exercise or routine becomes too challenging or monotonous, explore different options or modify your approach to keep it fresh and enjoyable.

13.4.4 Learn from Setbacks: View setbacks as learning experiences rather than failures. Use them as opportunities to reassess, adjust your approach, and move forward with renewed determination.

13.5 Tracking Progress:

Tracking your progress is crucial for maintaining motivation and recognizing your achievements. Consider the following methods for tracking progress:

13.5.1 Keep a Workout Journal: Document your workouts, noting the exercises, sets, reps, and any personal records. This allows you to track your progress and see improvements over time.

13.5.2 Take Measurements: Track your body measurements, such as weight, body fat percentage, and circumference measurements. Regularly reassessing these measurements will help you gauge progress.

13.5.3 Use Technology: Utilize fitness apps, wearable devices, or online platforms that allow you to track and monitor your workouts, nutrition, and progress.

13.5.4 Take Progress Photos: Capture progress photos periodically to visually see changes in your physique and compare them over time.

13.6 Embracing Flexibility:

Flexibility and adaptability are crucial in maintaining motivation. Consider the following strategies for embracing flexibility:

13.6.1 Be Realistic: Set realistic expectations and be flexible with your timeline. Recognize that progress takes time and that setbacks may occur.

13.6.2 Embrace Variety: Incorporate variety into your workouts by trying new exercises, exploring different fitness modalities, or challenging yourself with new goals. This prevents boredom and keeps your motivation high.

13.6.3 Adjust to Circumstances: Life can be unpredictable, and circumstances may require adjustments to your fitness routine. Embrace flexibility and find alternative ways to stay active and maintain consistency.

13.6.4 Be Kind to Yourself: Recognize that progress is not always linear, and there may be ups and downs along the way. Be kind to yourself and avoid being too hard on yourself when faced with obstacles or setbacks.

13.7 Seeking Inspiration:

Seeking inspiration can reignite your motivation and help you overcome challenging times. Consider the following techniques for finding inspiration:

13.7.1 Read Success Stories: Read success stories of individuals who have achieved similar goals to yours. Learn from their journeys, setbacks, and triumphs.

13.7.2 Follow Fitness Influencers: Follow fitness influencers, athletes, or professionals on social media who share their knowledge, experiences, and motivational content.

13.7.3 Engage in Mindful Activities: Engage in activities that inspire and uplift you, such as reading motivational books, listening to inspiring podcasts, or watching motivational videos.

13.7.4 Visualize Your Success: Spend time visualizing yourself achieving your goals. Think about how it will make you feel and the difference it will make in your life. This visualization can fuel your motivation and determination.

13.8 Celebrating Milestones:

Celebrating milestones along your fitness journey is essential for maintaining motivation and reinforcing your progress. Take into account the following strategies to recognize your accomplishments:

13.8.1 Set Milestone Rewards: Establish rewards for reaching specific milestones. Treat yourself to something you enjoy, such as a massage, a new workout outfit, or a day off to relax and rejuvenate.

13.8.2 Share Your Success: Share your achievements with your support system. Celebrate your milestones with friends and loved ones who can provide encouragement and celebrate with you.

13.8.3 Reflect and Appreciate: Take time to reflect on your progress and appreciate the hard work you've put in. Recognize the effort you've invested and the positive changes you've experienced.

13.8.4 Set New Goals: After celebrating a milestone, set new goals to continue challenging yourself and maintaining your motivation. Continually striving for progress keeps you engaged and inspired.

Conclusion:

Chapter 13 has addressed the critical aspect of staying motivated and overcoming obstacles in your home fitness journey. By setting clear goals, finding intrinsic motivation, building a support system, and developing strategies to overcome obstacles, you can stay on track and achieve your desired fitness outcomes. Embrace flexibility, track your progress, seek inspiration, and celebrate your milestones to maintain motivation and sustain a healthy and fulfilling fitness lifestyle. Remember, staying motivated is a continual process, and with determination, resilience, and the strategies outlined in this chapter, you can overcome challenges and achieve long-term success.

Chapter 14: Tracking Your Progress

Introduction:

In Chapter 14, we explore the importance of tracking your progress in your home fitness journey. Monitoring and measuring your progress is crucial for staying motivated, assessing the effectiveness of your efforts, and making necessary adjustments to achieve your fitness goals. This chapter will guide you through various methods and tools to effectively track and evaluate your progress, allowing you to make informed decisions and maintain momentum in your fitness journey.

14.1 Why Track Your Progress:

Tracking your progress provides several benefits in your fitness journey:

14.1.1 Motivation and Accountability: Seeing tangible evidence of your progress can boost motivation, reminding you of how far you've come and encouraging you to keep pushing forward.

14.1.2 Assessing Effectiveness: Tracking allows you to evaluate the effectiveness of your workout routines, nutrition choices, and lifestyle habits. This insight enables you to make adjustments to optimize your progress.

14.1.3 Identifying Plateaus and Adjustments: Plateaus are common in any fitness journey. By tracking your progress, you can identify periods of stagnation and take appropriate measures to overcome them.

14.1.4 Setting Realistic Goals: Regularly tracking your progress helps you set realistic and achievable goals based on your individual capabilities and progress rate.

14.1.5 Celebrating Achievements: Tracking provides a tangible way to celebrate milestones and accomplishments, reinforcing your dedication and boosting confidence.

14.2 What to Track:

Consider tracking the following aspects of your fitness journey:

14.2.1 Body Measurements: Record measurements such as weight, body fat percentage, waist circumference, and other relevant body measurements. These measurements reflect changes in body composition and help assess progress beyond just the number on the scale.

14.2.2 Strength and Endurance: Track your strength and endurance by recording the weights, reps, and sets you to perform for various exercises. Note any improvements or increases in performance over time.

14.2.3 Fitness Assessments: Conduct periodic fitness assessments, such as timed runs, maximum push-ups or squats, flexibility tests, or cardiovascular endurance tests. Compare your results to previous assessments to gauge improvements.

14.2.4 Workout Logs: Keep a detailed workout log, documenting the exercises, sets, reps, rest periods, and any additional notes about the intensity or difficulty level. This log provides a comprehensive overview of your training sessions.

14.2.5 Nutrition and Food Diary: Track your daily food intake by maintaining a food diary. Record the types of foods consumed, portion sizes, and any relevant nutritional information. This helps evaluate your dietary choices and identify areas for improvement.

14.2.6 Energy and Mood: Consider tracking your energy levels, mood, and sleep quality. Notice how they fluctuate based on your exercise routine, nutrition, and overall lifestyle habits.

14.3 Tracking Methods and Tools:

Utilize the following methods and tools to track your progress effectively:

14.3.1 Pen and Paper: Traditional methods such as using a notebook or journal can be effective for tracking progress. Create designated sections for each aspect you want to monitor, and update them regularly.

14.3.2 Mobile Apps: Numerous fitness and health tracking apps are available, allowing you to conveniently log and track various aspects of your fitness journey. These apps often offer features like progress charts, goal setting, and reminders.

14.3.3 Wearable Devices: Consider using wearable devices such as fitness trackers or smartwatches that monitor metrics like steps taken, heart rate, and calories burned. These devices provide real-time data and can sync with apps or online platforms for comprehensive tracking.

14.3.4 Online Platforms: Online platforms and websites dedicated to fitness tracking and community support can provide comprehensive tools to monitor your progress. They often offer features like progress graphs, challenges, and forums for interaction with like-minded individuals.

14.4 Frequency of Tracking:

The frequency of tracking may vary based on personal preferences and goals. Consider the following approaches:

14.4.1 Daily or Weekly Tracking: Some individuals prefer to track their progress daily or weekly to maintain a detailed record and closely monitor changes.

14.4.2 Periodic Tracking: Others may choose to track progress on a monthly or quarterly basis. This approach allows for a broader perspective of long-term progress and minimizes the potential stress associated with daily tracking.

14.4.3 Combination Approach: You can combine both approaches by tracking specific aspects, such as workout performance or body measurements, more frequently while assessing overall progress periodically.

14.5 Analyzing and Using Your Progress Data:

Once you have tracked your progress, it's essential to analyze and use the data to inform your fitness journey. Consider the following:

14.5.1 Set New Goals: Evaluate your progress and set new goals based on the data. Ensure these goals are specific, measurable, achievable, relevant, and time-bound (SMART goals).

14.5.2 Identify Patterns and Trends: Look for patterns and trends in your progress data. Identify what factors contribute to positive changes and what may hinder progress. Use this information to make informed decisions about adjustments in your routine or habits.

14.5.3 Seek Professional Guidance: If you're uncertain about interpreting your progress data or making necessary adjustments, consider consulting a fitness professional or registered dietitian. They can provide expert guidance and help you develop an effective plan based on your progress and goals.

14.5.4 Celebrate Milestones: Recognize and celebrate milestones along your fitness journey. Use the progress data to reflect on achievements and reward yourself for the dedication and hard work you've put in.

Conclusion:

Chapter 14 has emphasized the importance of tracking your progress in your home fitness journey. By monitoring and evaluating your progress, you can stay motivated, assess the effectiveness of your efforts, and make necessary adjustments to achieve your fitness goals. Whether you choose to track body measurements, strength, endurance, nutrition, or other aspects, use the methods and tools that work best for you. Remember to analyze and utilize your progress data to set new goals, identify patterns, seek professional guidance when needed, and celebrate your achievements along the way. Tracking your progress provides valuable insights that empower you to make informed decisions and maintain momentum in your fitness journey.

CONCLUSION

Congratulations! You have reached the end of this comprehensive guide, "Get Fit at Home." We hope this book has provided you with valuable insights, practical advice, and the motivation you need to embark on a successful home fitness journey. By exploring various topics, from understanding the benefits of home fitness to incorporating yoga, strength training, and nutrition into your routine, you now have a solid foundation to achieve your fitness goals.

We sincerely thank you for choosing this book as your guide. We understand that your commitment to improving your health and fitness is an important investment of your time and energy. We hope that the knowledge and tools shared in this book have empowered you to take control of your well-being and embrace the convenience and effectiveness of home workouts.

As you progress in your fitness journey, we encourage you to keep track of your achievements, overcome obstacles, and stay motivated.

Remember to celebrate your successes, no matter how small, and maintain a positive mindset. Consistency and determination will lead you to the desired results.

We kindly ask you to take a moment to leave a positive review for this book. Your feedback will not only help us improve future editions but also assist other readers in making informed decisions about their fitness journey. Your support is greatly appreciated.

Now, armed with the knowledge and inspiration gained from this book, it's time for you to take the first step or continue your journey toward a healthier and fitter you. Embrace the convenience of exercising at home, follow the principles of nutrition, listen to your body, and never forget the importance of rest and recovery.

Remember, this is not just a temporary endeavor but a lifelong commitment to your health and well-being. Stay consistent, adapt when needed, and enjoy the process. Your efforts will yield long-lasting benefits that extend far beyond physical fitness.

Thank you once again for choosing "Get Fit at Home." We wish you every success on your fitness journey and a life filled with vitality, strength, and happiness.

Stay motivated, stay committed, and embrace the transformative power of home fitness!

With gratitude,

[J. B. Blackwood]